The Effectiveness of a Vaccine for HIV: How Close Are We to the End of the Epidemic?

Michael A. Capristo

B.S.B.A., Stevens-Henager College, 2014

Submitted in Partial Fulfillment
of the Requirements for the Degree of
Masters of Science in Healthcare Administration

Independence University
May 2015

Approval Page

INDEPENDENCE UNIVERSITY

As members of the Final Project Committee, we certify that we have read the

document prepared by

Michael A. Capristo

entitled

The Effectiveness of a Vaccine for HIV: How Close Are We to the End of the Epidemic?

and recommend that it be accepted as fulfilling the final project requirement for the

Degree of

Masters of Science in Healthcare Administration

*Dr. Doret Ledford*_____ Date: 4/30/2015_____
Name of Course Instructor

_____Date: ___04/30/2015_____
Dr. Carmen Spears, Dean of Health Science

Abstract

The Effectiveness of a Vaccine for HIV: How Close Are We to the End of the Epidemic?

Michael A. Capristo

Submitted in partial fulfillment of the requirements for the

Degree of

Masters of Science in Healthcare Administration

Independence University

May 2015

Abstract

This thesis examined the HIV and AIDS pandemic; its history, research into likely genetic lineage, mutations and species crossover. This work included review of recent literature, studies and clinical research which were aimed at understanding HIV/AIDS in order to develop methods of infection prevention including; education, vaccine and genetic modification strategies. Increasing numbers of studies, trials and clinical research have been gaining recognition and provided insightful knowledge of groundbreaking approaches to fighting HIV and AIDS. To explore how the combination of recent research breakthroughs might affect the fight against the pandemic going forward, this thesis analyzed numerous literature sources and studies.

Dedication

I wish to dedicate this work to the three most important people in my life. Without their support this work would not have been possible. First my mother Paula Capristo who taught me the value of family, ethics, responsibility, the meaning of unconditional love, always provided unwavering support, unequaled advice and encouragement beyond words. Thank you for my life, for being my Rock of Gibraltar during life's storms, and for being my best friend always. My sister, Jennifer Capristo Ingram who has shown time and again that super heroines really do exist and made having courage, conviction, unimpeachable character, grace, beauty and intelligence all look easy. If it were not for these two unimaginably strong, graceful, beautiful and articulate women, I would have never completed college. Finally, for my partner, Dave Houck who has supported me in every way a person can through this journey. You have encouraged me, supported me when I felt I couldn't go on, consoled me when I felt defeated and celebrated with me when I reached goals. Dave, I will always remember your words, "They don't just give away Masters Degrees". This milestone I dedicate to these people because I am who I am through them.

I love you always, always, always.

Acknowledgements

It is with the greatest of gratitude that I acknowledge Ms. Terrie Jenkins who acted as my Associate Dean of Student Services through both my Bachelors and Master's Degree programs. Thank you for coming to my rescue when I needed you, always patiently listening, being incredibly supportive, for being my friend and confidante through my academic journey. I would also like to thank Dr. Doret Ledford for her unwavering and inspiring positivity, bold confidence and sound editorial advice throughout the writing process of this document. My favorite quote from her which I will carry for the rest of my days; "Let us all strive to do better". To all of my esteemed Professors and Dr. Alan Hansen, Executive Director, it has been the greatest privilege of my life to learn from you. My knowledge has been greatly increased through your patience, efforts and wisdom…for which I will be eternally grateful.

Table of Contents

List of Tables

Chapter 1: Introduction

Since the onslaught and spread of the Human Immuno-deficiency Virus (HIV) was discovered, researchers have been feverishly searching for a vaccine and a cure to end the deadly epidemic. The most recent United Nations statistics indicate that "Approximately 39 million people have died from HIV related illnesses since the epidemic began in 1981" ("UNAIDS fact sheet", 2015). As published in the New England Journal of Medicine; "it is a global priority for researchers to find an efficacious and viable vaccine to fight HIV" (Hammer, Sobieszcyk, Magdalena, et al, 2013). This paper will provide a conceptual framework regarding how the epidemic began and subsequently flourished in the United States and will include aspects of politics, social elements and healthcare industry specific facts that all played into the development of the disease within society. The progression of clinical research and understanding of the disease will also be related. It is widely accepted that the HIV epidemic has claimed millions of lives worldwide, although the actual number of deaths is impossible to accurately calculate. One study in South Africa successfully demonstrated that "misclassified deaths across fourteen other disease categories between 1996 and 2006 revealed the reported 19% HIV/AIDS related deaths was actually 48% (with an uncertainty percentage between 7-28%)" (Birnbaum, Murray & Lozano, 2011). Vigorous research has provided dramatic improvements in treatment regime protocols that have translated into positive patient outcomes. These positive outcomes can be seen in the treatment of HIV patients who also have an opportunistic infection such as pneumocystis pneumonia (PCP); "…advanced and extremely active medication protocol improvements have dramatically reduced the occurrence of PCP in patients in industrialized nations" (Tachikawa, Tomii, Murase &Ueda, et al, 2011). Efforts in research have focused on finding an effective vaccine and recent discoveries are providing the hope of a cure for those already infected.

Background

Thirty-four years ago a worldwide pandemic began as an epidemic in The United States. At that time; "it was referred to as Gay Related Immune Deficiency (GRID) syndrome; the disease we know today as Human Immunodeficiency Virus/Acquired Immune Deficiency Syndrome (HIV/AIDS)" (Lovell & Rosenberg, 2011). From the very beginning of the epidemic those affected have been asking the same question; "When will this be over?" Clinicians, researchers, patients and advocates are still asking that question. Because of research efforts and activism today we better understand the disease and are more educated about HIV and AIDS. There is less societal stigmatization, more compassion, increased visibility and acceptance of those affected. A vast research machine is striving to bring a solution to the problem of HIV/AIDS through science. According to the American Public Health Association (APHA); "HIV/AIDS is the single largest health issue that has changed the landscape of the modern era with broad social impact" (Stover & Northridge, 2013). The effort in the battle against HIV/AIDS is two fold; preventing the spread of additional infection (likely by perfecting a vaccine) and elimination of the disease in already infected persons.

In order to understand where we are today (and our likely path forward) in the fight against HIV/AIDS we must first understand the most probable origins and progression of the disease. In 1981 the social climate in The United States was fervently intolerant of homosexuality. In fact, the stigmatization of homosexuality during this period in time was a huge contributing factor to the spread of HIV/AIDS. "The stigma attached to both HIV positive status and homosexuality are both obstacles to effective HIV prevention" (Bird & Voisin, 2013). Institutionalized discrimination of the homosexual community was common in both government and society at large. For example, in spite of being urged by the Centers for Disease Control (CDC) health officials to publicly address the issue, President Ronald Reagan refused to even comment on the spreading health emergency. This silence from the White House lasted for over seven years and over 30,000 American citizens died of the disease in the interim. "In spite of explicit and early documentation regarding the threat posed by HIV/AIDS, the Reagan Administration refused to implement programs and provide funding to prevent further spread of the disease within American society" (Francis, 2012). This inaction prevented desperately needed deployment of emergency health plans, services and funding that would have likely helped to stem the spread of the disease during this period of time.

In direct response to political apathy, social disdain and discrimination, the Gay Rights Movement gained momentum. This simultaneously provided needed visibility and support to help fight HIV and AIDS. "The importance of the gay community's participation in fighting HIV/AIDS; is impossible to deny" (Zablotska, Holt & Prestage, 2011). Outspoken proponents for research included most notably actresses and philanthropists Elizabeth Taylor and Doris Day; both of whom lost friend and fellow actor Rock Hudson to the disease. Among others, these celebrities lent their voices and visibility to those affected by HIV/AIDS. At the time those affected by the disease were so stigmatized that they were virtually invisible and isolated. Their activism efforts focused on motivating political and social shifts to bring about awareness and funding for research. Piers Morgan commenting for CNN news regarding Elizabeth Taylor's HIV activism, "She was among the first to speak out on behalf of people living with HIV when others reacted with fear and often outright hostility" (France, 2011). To date there is virtually no segment of global society that has been left untouched by the disease of HIV/AIDS.

Statement of the Problem

"The problem of HIV and AIDS is a worldwide pandemic that, to-date, has lasted over thirty years" (Sharp & Hahn, 2011). Currently there are two world populations; those who are infected with HIV and those who are not. In order to prevent future infections an effective vaccine to prevent transmission must be perfected, manufactured in mass, and be disseminated for immunizations around the world. In order to eliminate HIV from those already infected an effective means of eradicating the virus in a living person must also be perfected.

Research Questions

The research questions are;

1. Will a vaccine for HIV effectively prevent the transmission of HIV?

2. Are there any new research discoveries that could potentially be used to eliminate HIV from an infected person?

3. If the first two questions prove positive, will the combination of the two answers effectively end the HIV epidemic?

Hypotheses

From these questions the following hypotheses are created;

$H1_a$: Those vaccinated for HIV are more likely to become infected with HIV.

$H1_0$: Those vaccinated for HIV are less likely to become infected with HIV.

$H2_a$: It is likely that there are new research discoveries that could potentially be utilized to eliminate HIV from a person already infected.

$H2_0$: It is not likely that there are new research discoveries that could potentially be utilized to eliminate HIV from a person already infected.

$H3_a$: If the answers to the first two questions prove positive, the combination of the two is likely to effectively end the HIV epidemic.

$H3_0$: If the answers to the first two questions prove positive, the combination of the two is unlikely to effectively end the HIV epidemic.

Basic Assumptions and Limitations

Some of the basic assumptions for this paper include;

- Researchers are both actively pursuing an effective vaccine for HIV;

- Researchers are engaged in efforts to discover an effective means of eliminating HIV from an already infected person;

- It is possible to mass produce a vaccine for HIV

- If and when discovered, the cost of that production is feasible and worldwide dissemination is also possible.

Limitations include the fact that it is not possible to determine when future discoveries will be made or how effective or useful they will be regarding treatment or elimination of HIV. An additional limiting factor would be adherence to any type of vaccination and/or treatment protocol for either the prevention of transmission or the eradication of HIV from an already infected person. As the news has highly publicized, many people remain skeptical of the safety of vaccines. As such any individuals who choose to remain unvaccinated would theoretically remain at risk.

Definitions of Terms

Acquired Immune-deficiency Syndrome – also known as AIDS, this is the group of clinical diseases that, together, can be attributed to HIV infection.

Allele – several types of genes that are typically created through the process of mutation which are the basis for hereditary variation.

Antiretroviral Therapy – also known as ART, is the combination of medications used to treat human immune deficiency virus infection in humans. In most patients this treatment protocol is a combination of three classes of drugs.

Booster – a drug administered to increase the power of another or to expand the intended capability of a companion medication

CCR5Δ32 – C-C chemokine receptor type 5 gene with 32-bp deletions occur in patients that possess natural resistance to infection by HIV.

CD4 – these are the primary cells of the human immune system which are used to fight infection. These cells are also the primary target of the HIV virus.

Centers for Disease Control – also known as the CDC, is The United States leading governmental agency for the prevention and protection of citizens from disease.

Clinical Trial Phases – the stages (or steps) of moving a proposed drug or treatment further in the approval process for widespread use. Each of the stages is designed to provide a response to a research question. There are four phases of human trials;

Phase I – administered to a small number of people to evaluate safety, side effects and effective dosage.

Phase II – administered to a larger group (than phase I) to further evaluate effectiveness and safety.

Phase III – administered to large groups of people (plural) to confirm prior findings of effectiveness, side effects, compare to other known treatments and procure other data which provides for safety in future use.

Phase IV – studies conducted post marketing regarding the drug or treatment's effect(s) on various populations, including potential long-term side effects not previously detected.

Cluster Regularly Interspaced Short Palindromic Repeats – also known as CRISPR, is a newly discovered technology that is derived from bacteria's ability to protect itself from viral infections; currently still in research phase of development.

CRISPR/Cas9 – CRISPR associated proteins (Cas9) that degrade sequences of HIV which inhibits viral infiltration of CD4 (immune system) cells.

Diphtheria – a preventable infection (via vaccination) that causes a thick coating in the back of the throat; as a result arrested breathing, cardiac arrest and death can occur.

ELISA – acronym for Enzyme Linked Immuno-sorbent Assay, which is the predominantly used and preferred test for HIV due to its sensitivity to HIV related antibodies.

Epidemic – a disease that, although geographically widespread, is limited to one continent or region.

Food and Drug Administration – also known as the FDA, is The United States federal governmental agency that regulates ingestible and topical substances; food and medications must be approved by this agency before distribution to the public.

Gay Related Immune Deficiency – also known as GRID, a phrase originally coined in the early 1980's prior to the isolation and identification of the human immune-deficiency virus.

Hepatitis – inflammation of the liver; there are five different types (A-E) of which there is a vaccine for both A and B.

Highly Active Antiretroviral Therapy – also known as HAART, is the combination of three classes of drugs used to treat the human immune deficiency virus. This term is interchangeably used with the more abbreviated term antiretroviral therapy (ART).

Human Immune-deficiency Virus – also known as HIV, is the virus that causes acquired immune deficiency syndrome disease (AIDS).

Induced Pluripotent Stem Cells – also known as iPSCs, are pluripotent stem cells which can be propagated directly from mature cells.

Long Terminal Repeats – also known as LTR, are identical repeating sequences of genetic retroviral material which are used by viruses to insinuate themselves into host genomes.

Pandemic – an epidemic that has spread to two or more continents.

Pertussis – also known as Whooping Cough is a preventable disease (via vaccination) that can cause arrested breathing in babies.

Phase I, II, III or IV – see Clinical Trial Phases

PiggyBac – also known as PiggyBac (PB) transposon is a mobile genetic element that allows the cutting and pasting of chromosomal sites which has been highly effective in genetic engineering and modification sciences.

Pluripotent – **a** descriptive term for the ability of a cell to develop into any type of specifically purposed cell; with the exception of embryonic or placenta cells.

Polymerase Chain Reaction – a technological process in biological research that is used to effectively replicate a small quantity of DNA copies into a much larger sample.

Proviral/Provirus – a virus that is fully integrated into the DNA of its host.

Puromycin – a selective antibiotic agent used in research to kill all cells that are not puromycin resistant; provides researchers a means to create a "clean" culture.

Reservoirs – areas of the body where latent (dormant) HIV resides within the body of an infected person. These areas are still being identified by researchers. One reservoir that has been identified is fluid surrounding the human brain.

Retrovirus/Retroviral – the family of viruses which replicate via the process of reverse transcription. As an RNA based (with a DNA intermediate), once it invades a host cell it uses its own reverse transcriptase enzyme in order to manufacture DNA from the viral RNA (which is in reverse pattern meaning retro); the viral DNA is inserted into the host cell genome which is then called a provirus.

RV144 – also known as the Thai HIV efficacy trial was an HIV effectiveness trial conducted by the United States Military in Thailand on strains of the virus commonly found in that region of the world. RV144 was a combination of two vaccines; one a primary and the other a boost (engineered to make the former more effective).

Transcription Activator-Like Effector Nucleases – also known as TALENS genetically modified enzymes created to cleave DNA at a precise location on the strand. This allows for the introduction of other genetically modified material into the DNA sequence.

Tetanus – also known as Lockjaw, is a bacteria based infection which is not transmittable from person to person rather it is acquired through open skin (cuts, tears or punctures) with contaminated objects such as rusty metal, soil or fecal matter.

Vaccine/Vaccination – the introduction of dead virus biological preparations or other agents scientifically designed to trigger the immune system to produce antibodies in order to provide protection from disease.

Conclusion

Once research revealed that AIDS was caused by a virus (HIV), many researchers came to the conclusion that a vaccine must be developed because that is the tactic which worked in so many previous disease battles. "Historically, vaccines have been our best weapon against the world's deadliest infectious diseases including; smallpox, polio, measles, and yellow fever" ("HIV vaccine research", 2015). Many diseases have been either controlled or eliminated from the human population through the proper, effective administration of vaccination programs and protocols. Additionally, many of these diseases are virus based including polio; the vaccine for which was discovered by Dr. Jonas Salk in the 1950's. Other successful vaccines that are approved by the Food and Drug Administration (FDA) include; Tetanus, Pertussis, Diphtheria and Hepatitis A and B. In this same regard, researchers have been searching for a vaccine that will be effective in fighting HIV. Other methods for HIV prevention, i.e. advocation of abstinence from unprotected sexual activity, discouraging promiscuity and efforts to thwart intravenous drug users from sharing contaminated needles, have yielded mediocre results at best.

Discoveries are emerging that are expected to prove valuable in being able to perfect a viable method to eliminate HIV from an already infected individual. New biotechnology discoveries, such as Cluster Regularly Interspaced Short Palindromic Repeats (CRISPR) technology [see Definitions of Terms above], has proven effective in allowing researchers to eliminate viruses and genetic abnormalities which cause disease. CRISPR technology, although some time away from human trials, has shown to be effective in animal testing thus far.

The development of both a vaccine and a viable method to eradicate HIV from an infected person may very well prove to be the tipping point that brings about the much awaited end to the pandemic of HIV and AIDS.

Due to the global characteristic of the HIV/AIDS pandemic there is a wealth of published, scholarly literature on the subject from a variety of research specialties. Additionally, because thirty-four years have passed since the identification of the virus there have been many studies, clinical trials of medications and vaccines that have been documented in the literature. Documentation of the likely lineage of the pathogen itself and the history of the pandemic are also well recounted in literature.

Chapter 2: Literature Review

Overview

As of 2013 approximately thirty-nine million people have died as a result of HIV infection and an additional thirty-five million are infected worldwide (Hosein, 2015). The battle against HIV and AIDS has been one of the primary focuses of researchers for over thirty years (Lahey, 2015; Avert, 2015). The initial emergence and discovery of the disease coincided with a period in history when the gay population was generally vilified, reviled and shunned. This attitude contributed to a woefully inadequate response from the healthcare infrastructure (Avert, 2015).

Traditional approaches to fighting this disease included the development of medications to manage the infection essentially transforming it into a chronic condition (in developed nations) rather than the death sentence the diagnosis was during the early years of the epidemic (Avert, 2015). However, "In spite of the development of over thirty medications that have demonstrated complete suppression of the virus's replication ability progression of the disease remains a problem" (Bernstein, 2015). Researchers at the Doudna Lab at University of California at Berkeley contend that recent scientific developments in the genetic therapy arena have given them the hope of being able to eradicate the virus from an already infected individual (Doudna, 2015). Laurence, et al., 2015 asserts that, pharmaceutical and biotechnology breakthroughs have for the first time forced dormant HIV out of 'safe harbor' reservoirs making them vulnerable to treatment and possibly even eradication from the body. These reservoirs, such as those identified in the human brain, are areas where HIV can remain dormant and invulnerable to current medications. Additional research which has proven successful is a gene therapy based treatment that renders the HIV in a person's body harmless, while it "does not eradicate the disease researchers are classifying this discovery as a functional cure" (Kempner, 2015).

It is well known that the availability of literature recounting the history of the epidemic, from a plethora of perspectives, within the borders of the United States as well as around the world is plentiful and well-documented. There is also a wealth of literature documenting entire bodies of work, including the most likely genetic lineage of HIV, transmission events (including cross-species), medications and treatments (Sharp & Hahn, 2011). There are some literary works beginning to appear that highlight new, groundbreaking discoveries that for the first time probe how to eradicate HIV from reservoirs within the body where the virus has remained dormant and invulnerable to known treatments ("The Body Pro", 2015; Marlett, et al., 2015; Jungwirth, 2015; Ebina, et al., 2013). Additional groundbreaking research is appearing in the literature describing yet more groups of researchers who are working on eradicating the disease in already infected individuals through genetic therapies (Jungwirth, 2015; Ebina, et al., 2013).

As exciting and encouraging as all of these individual discoveries are; there is virtually no literature available that asserts how the combination of these innovations is likely to impact the fight against HIV and AIDS. Several of the research breakthroughs have only appeared in literature within the last few months (for example, Researchers Doudna and Fauci); a possible reason that no literature is available regarding the effect(s) the combination of discoveries will provide.

Although the advancements in the science of HIV continue to be very different and unique; their mutual goal is the same, to provide a piece to the greater puzzle of understanding and ultimately conquering HIV. The following will review literature regarding;

- How the Epidemic Began

- Prevention of HIV through Treatment of Infected Patients

- HIV Vaccine Development

- Elimination of the Disease in Persons Already Infected

- The Difference between Curing HIV and Curing AIDS.

How the Epidemic Began

AVERT: History of AIDS Up to 1986

This chronology of the pandemic shows there were unknown numbers of cases prior to 1980. According to Jonathan Mann (2014), "the spread of HIV had already reached a minimum of five separate continents by 1980 and approximately 100,000-300,000 people were likely already infected". The chronology continues through each year through 1986, documenting the typical symptoms of patients, their locations and quoting numerous eye witnesses to the beginning of the HIV epidemic. Events such as the 1984 press conference in which Health and Human Services Secretary Margaret Heckler, alongside Dr. Robert Gallo of the National Cancer Institute, declared they had found the cause of AIDS and that a test was soon to be available to detect the virus. They also announced (incorrectly) their estimate of two years for a vaccine to be developed and available to the public (Avert, 2015).

Although AVERT cites a wealth of statistical data from around the world regarding the evolution of the disease, it omits depth in realistically describing the political and social perspectives of the early 1980's pertaining to HIV/AIDS. Due to this omission, this work does not provide a full scope of the harsh reality the public, and more specifically the homosexual community, was faced with from 1980 through 1986.

Origins of HIV and the AIDS Pandemic

The Origins of HIV and the AIDS Pandemic (2015), is a retrospective which provides the lineage of the likely origins of the pathogen HIV; citing the closely related Symbian Immunodeficiency Virus (SIV) and the cross-species transmission. This retrospective also maps the genetic mutations that presumably occurred from one species of Symbian to another and finally to humans as HIV. According to authors Sharp and Hahn (2011), the HIV-1 pandemic is not a single virus but rather four separate strains (M, N, O and P) all of which originated and can be traced to original host species of chimpanzees, apes and gorillas in the southeastern Cameroon region of Africa. This work authoritatively established the likely origins and routes of transmission events which lead to the pandemic we know today. This retrospective provided a critical foundational structure for understanding the likely origination points and mutation pathways into human beings, a scientific cornerstone for genetic HIV research today.

Prevention of HIV through Treatment of Infected Patients

New Lead against HIV Could Finally Hobble the Virus's Edge

The journal publication from Medicalxpress dated March 18, 2015, describes the research and findings of Dr. Dennis Liotta and his colleagues at Emory University. Traditional medications designed to treat HIV have targeted a single action or behavior of the virus. However, Dr. Liotta and his team have adopted a new approach; developing a single drug which addresses the disease replication process at several different stages while at the same time minimizing the drug's side effects. This drug is also very inexpensive to manufacture in comparison to current medications which are notoriously expensive to produce (Bernstein, 2015).

The HIV Treatment Cascade-A new Tool in HIV Prevention

According to Dr. Thomas Giordano in the Journal of the American Medical Association (JAMA); the cascade of care, or the steps in the continuum of care, for newly diagnosed HIV patients is having incredible impact on the continuation of the pandemic (2015). Dr. Giordano relates that specific activities must happen if care is to be effective. The steps that he prescribes as necessary are; infected individuals must be diagnosed, they must engage in care, antiretroviral therapy (ART) must commence, and they must adhere to treatment regimens and regular physician visits. In his commentary Dr. Giordano asserts that in 2005, 26% of patients achieved viral suppression and in 2011 that percentage had only grown to 30%; an increase of four percentage points in six years. Dr. Giordano attributed this slow growth in the rate of viral suppression directly to the lack of implementation of the cascade of care. He goes on to cite both delay of diagnosis and poor retention in care and adherence as primary factors that result in nearly 90% of new disease transmissions in the U.S (Giordano, 2015).

The relevance of this work is tremendous according to researchers with the Centers for Disease Control in Atlanta. Researcher Giordano summarizes the impact of poor implementation of the cascade of care on his study population. Steps that are not happening in the continuum of care are perpetuating the pandemic such as; poor early diagnosis rates, consistent ART treatment adherence and lack of engagement in care. He further clarifies that if the cascade of care is not widely implemented there will likely be negative consequences including perpetuation of the disease.

Antiretroviral treatment of HIV-1 Prevents Transmission of HIV-1: Where do we go from here?

As published in medical journal The Lancet (2013); Myron S. Cohen, M. Kumi Smith, Kathryn E. Muessig, Timothy B. Hallett, Kimberly A. Powers, and Angela D. Kashuba relate that the HPTN 052 randomized controlled study demonstrated that HIV transmission is reduced by 96.4% when both ART and condoms are utilized in tandem. Additionally noted is that a pool of evidence is expanding which indicates that early treatment with medication may possibly curb HIV presence within the general population. If these results are to be realized outside of controlled trial conditions two requirements would need to be met. These requirements would be that ART be universally available and the adherence percentages would also need to be consistently high (Cohen, et al., 2013).

HIV Vaccine Development

RV144 Clinical Trial

The U.S. Military HIV Research Program (MHRP) clinical trial of RV144 [see Definition of Terms], also known as the Thai HIV vaccine efficacy trial sponsored by the U.S. Army Surgeon General, completed their study in 2013 on the efficacy of the compound in phase III trials. In a phase III trial the medication is administered to a large number of people to assess; effectiveness, side effects and safety. RV144 was thought to be effective against specific virus strains common to this region of the world. The clinical trials were located in Rayong and Chon Buri Provinces, Thailand, according to the report from the MHRP (2015).

Why HIV Vaccines May Be Failing

According to author, consultant and sexual health expert Martha Kempner in The Body Pro: The HIV Resource for Health Professionals (2015); a vaccine for HIV has been elusive because HIV is unique in that it targets immune cells that traditional vaccines utilize in order to create immunity. Ms. Kempner goes on to assert that recent research has demonstrated that immune response prompted by an HIV derived vaccine may actually increase the likelihood of transmission.

New Paradigms for HIV/AIDS Vaccine Development

This research report by the U.S. National Library of Medicine: National Institutes of Health in the Annual Review of Medicine described HIV's unique ability to protect itself. Researchers Picker, Hansen and Lifson (2013), assert that both HIV-1 and its simian relative SIV are uniquely adapted to prevent immunity in their host. The primary discussion of the authors revolves around the premise that the virus is particularly vulnerable to immunity during the early stages of infection and this vulnerability should be exploited for vaccine development purposes. They also contend that virus replication, once infection is established, occurs indefinitely. They observed that the combination of rapid mutation and replication of HIV has proven problematic for vaccine development. The authors also detail the virus's unique ability to be able to prevent vaccine effectiveness due to its ability to quickly mutate; rendering the vaccines useless due to their specific strain focus.

New Approach to Blocking HIV Raises Hopes for an AIDS Vaccine

As reported by McNeil Jr. in The New York Times (2015), researchers including Dr. Anthony Fauci and Michael Farzan, asserted that this new gene modification treatment has been so successful at blocking HIV in animal trials that it could very well be a functional vaccine against AIDS. Researchers contend that this new technique splices genetic material into a very small strand of DNA which (when injected) triggers production of antibody-like proteins. According to the report these proteins effectively prevent HIV from entering cells. In spite of this encouraging news, Dr. Fauci remains reticent to proclaim victory citing that testing remains only in animal models and evidence must be produced that it is just as effective in humans. Michael Farzan of the Scripps Research Institute classified this discovery as the "most potent entry inhibitor" that has been identified to-date (McNeil, 2015).

Elimination of the Disease in Patients Already Infected

New Kick and Kill HIV Cure Drug, TLR7 Agonist, Shows Promise

According to The Body Pro: The HIV Resource for Healthcare Professionals (2015); a brand new classification of drug was unveiled at this year's Conference on Retroviruses and Opportunistic Infections (CROI) held in Seattle, Washington in February 2015. This medication, called a toll-like receptor 7 (TLR7) agonist, was for the first time capable of activating dormant HIV infected cells causing them to begin replication of the virus. Gilead Pharmaceuticals, the developer of TLR7, asserts that the drug is effective in activating latent HIV into activity thus making it vulnerable to treatment. Gilead asserts that, due to the fact that current ART treatments can only attack and kill active HIV cells, this is a huge breakthrough that has promising potential because it prevents virus latency.

Cellular Scissors Chop up HIV Virus

According to researchers at the Salk Institute; John Marlett, Juan Belmonte, Hsin-Kai Liao, Yuta Takahashi, Concepcion Esteban and Tomoaki Hishida (2015), they are on their way to creating a single medication that could not only prevent HIV infection but also treat those already infected and eradicate all dormant and hiding virus in the human body through the adaptation of Cluster Regularly Interspaced Short Palindromic Repeats (CRISPR), the molecular defense ability of bacteria against viruses [see Definition of Terms]. According to researchers, they are extremely excited about this discovery and are confident that CRISPR will erase the virus from the human genome. Although the Salk Institute researchers are admittedly encouraged by the discovery they estimate that more research is required to ascertain how the biotechnology might be used effectively and safely in human patients.

New HIV Gene Therapy Shows Promise in Mice

Author Barbara Jungwirth of The Body Pro: The HIV Resource for Health Professionals (2015) asserts that researchers have been able to recreate the functional cure of HIV experienced by "The Berlin Patient", Mr. Timothy Brown. According to Jungwirth, a study based out of the University of California, Davis was able to recreate the results in a mouse and the results have been published in the journal Stem Cells. According to researchers Barclay, Yang, Zhang, Fong, Barraza, Nolta…Anderson (2015), genetically engineered human stem cells were altered to be resistant to HIV. The HIV resistant stem cells were then implanted in mice. The researchers then exposed the mice to HIV which remained HIV test negative and healthy. Also according to researchers; previous genetic work in this arena was a failure with only a 17.5% immunity rate as opposed to the rate they are now able to achieve, which is 94.2% effective at replicating HIV resistant cells.

Harnessing the CRISPR/Cas9 System to Disrupt Latent HIV-1 Provirus

Researchers Ebina, Misawa, Kanemura and Koyanagi (2013) report that in spite of highly active antiretroviral therapy (HAART) ability to kill active HIV cells the virus is still able to remain dormant within hidden reservoirs [see Definition of Terms] in the body. According to researchers these dormant cells can activate and re-emerge at any time to begin replication and pose a pathogenic threat to the host. CRISPR/Cas9 [see Definition of Terms] biotechnology is not only able to seek out and kill active virus, but also dormant HIV cells as well, effectively eradicating the virus from the host entirely. According to Ebina, et al., (2013) their study methods were; gRNA expression plasmid, virus, cell culture, TF and flow cytometry, establishment of latent form of LTIG-transduced Jurkat cells, integration-site analysis of latently integrated LTIG provirus, quantitative analysis of HIV DNA and statistical analysis.

The Difference between Curing HIV and Curing AIDS

British Columbia Researchers Examine Past and Future Directions in the HIV Epidemic

According to author Sean R. Hosein with the Canadian AIDS Treatment Information Exchange, as published in The Body Pro: The HIV Resource for Health Professionals; researchers at the British Columbia Centre for Excellence in HIV/AIDS (CfE) in Vancouver emphasize that in spite of the phrase "end of AIDS" being prevalently heard in recent years, there is a tremendous distinction between ending HIV and ending AIDS citing that these are actually two separate issues and remarkably unique degrees of complexity. The Canadian researchers assert that HIV is less complex than a diagnosis of AIDS, which requires not only HIV infection but also the presence of an opportunistic infection (Hosein, 2015).

Information Disconnects for People Infected With, or Affected by, HIV/AIDS in the United Kingdom

Based on accounts shared with authors Namuleme, Ford and Bath as published in Direct Research Journal of Social Science and Educational Studies (2015) even today many people lack even the most basic of knowledge regarding HIV and AIDS. According to the authors, real world knowledge continues to be very rudimentary in many areas due to a lack of education and an over-abundance of stigmatization. These authors also relate that people should be educated regarding the fact that a person can have HIV without having AIDS. They relate that all people with AIDS have HIV and they also state that this concept is challenging for many people to understand. They further elaborate that this leads to a lack of understanding that curing HIV and curing AIDS are two different subjects and, are in fact, not the same thing.

The End of AIDS: HIV Infection as a Chronic Disease

Professors Deeks, Lewin and Havlir as published in the journal The Lancet (2013) assert that the diagnosis of AIDS is no longer a primary threat to the health of those infected with the HIV. Rather toxicity issues surrounding long-term exposure to medication regimens are the central core issues in treatment today. The authors cite that as long as patients are adherent to treatment protocols their disease should be regarded as a chronic disease or condition. They concluded that a diagnosis of AIDS is not a foregone conclusion due to the availability and effectiveness of ART.

Conclusion

The resources from the literature have shown that scientific strides have been achieved in treatment protocols and the possibility of a vaccine for HIV. The breakthrough of CRISPR/Cas9 biotechnology could also play a crucial role in curing HIV and AIDS. It is important to remember that the medication/treatment pipeline is a long and arduous process that can take years and, as a result, we may not see some of the work presented in the literature in human trials for some time to come. The reality is that there needs to be an effective cascade of care which includes widespread, early diagnosis and treatment of HIV (Giordano, 2015). However, the above sampling of literature (in combination) demonstrates that there is a cascade of negative events that happens when we fail to diagnose, fail to treat, fail to retain patients and fail to educate about HIV. These negative events ultimately result in the perpetuation of the HIV pandemic. As a result, our best defense currently against HIV/AIDS is to foster testing, treatment, adherence and education.

However, according to some of the literature there are incredible discoveries that may very well answer the questions;

- Will a vaccine for HIV effectively prevent the transmission of HIV?
- Are there any new research discoveries that could be utilized to eliminate HIV from an infected person?

  And, if these first two questions prove positive;

- Will the combination of the two effectively end the HIV epidemic?

Answering these three questions may very well serve to bring about an end to HIV and AIDS. Although additional research still needs to be undertaken to find these answers, there is a great wealth of research that has already been completed as this sampling of literature demonstrates. Research can employ any number, or combination, of methodologies in the effort to derive useable information in the fight against HIV and AIDS.

Chapter 3: Methodology

Research Method

This paper utilized pre-existing studies and employed the mixed-method in order to extrapolate qualitative information. Three studies were included here in order to provide a framework regarding where the research community is, in direct relationship to the three key research questions;

1.   Will a vaccine for HIV effectively prevent the transmission of HIV?

2.   Are there any new potential research discoveries that could be utilized to eliminate HIV from a person already infected?

3.   If the answers to the first two questions prove to be yes, will the combination of the two effectively end the HIV epidemic?

Research Questions and Hypotheses

The hypotheses that are created by these questions are as follows;

H1a: Those vaccinated for HIV are more likely to become infected with HIV.

H10: Those vaccinated for HIV are less likely to become infected with HIV.

H2a: It is likely that there are new potential research discoveries that could be utilized to eliminate HIV from a person already infected.

H20: It is not likely that there are new potential research discoveries that could be utilized to eliminate HIV from a person already infected.

H3a: If the first two questions prove positive, the combination of the two is likely to effectively end the HIV epidemic.

H30: If the first two questions prove positive, the combination of the two is unlikely to effectively end the HIV epidemic.

Studies

Study One: Long-term follow-up (LTFU) of study participants from prophylactic HIV vaccine clinical trials in Africa (March, 2014)

Researchers Schmidt, Jaoko, Omosa-Manyonyi, Kaleebu, Mpendo, Nanvubya... Fast (2014) conducted this study focusing on follow-up of vaccine trials administered between 2001 and 2007 in Africa. The researchers sought to define long term effects of a potential vaccine on recipients. The study was facilitated by the International AIDS Vaccine Initiative (IAVI) and was comprised of seven phase I and II trial sets. Research scientists placed dual emphasis on safety and effectiveness of two potential vaccines. The double-blind study was conducted with volunteers who were both HIV negative and healthy. Two types of candidate vaccines were tested during this trial, plasmid DNA and viral vector based. The LTFU study assessed multiple health criteria as well as immune response persistence via monthly blood tests for six consecutive months. Participants completed a health questionnaire and, in addition to being tested for HIV, were also screened for residual immune response. There were 287 participants in the LFTU, of which ninety-three percent asserted that they were in acceptable health at their final appointment.

The study examined (by comparison) both placebo recipients as well as those who had received at least a single dose of one of the subject compounds. Health outcomes of the control group were compared to the recipient group to establish variance (Schmidt, et al., 2014).

Study Two: Seamless modification of wild-type induced pluripotent stem cells to the natural CCR5Δ32 mutation confers resistance to HIV infection (June, 2014)

Researchers Ye, Wang, Beyer, Teque, Cradick, Qi...Kan (2014) contend that the purpose of this study was to assess the feasibility, effectiveness and outcomes associated with combining two approaches, each of which provide HIV-1 immunity. This study also endeavored to recreate natural immunity to HIV-1 infection. The researchers sought to achieve this through manual genetic modification of stem cells utilizing both transcription activator-like effector nucleases (TALENS) or RNA targeted clustered regularly interspaced short palindromic repeats (CRISPR)-Cas9.

One premise this study operated under was the successful outcome of Timothy Brown, also known as The Berlin Patient, who was the first patient considered to have been cured of HIV-1 infection. This patient's extensive treatment for Leukemia included total bone marrow ablation and reintroduction of HIV-1 resistant CD4 cells. This effectively rebuilt his immune system incorporating HIV immunity against future infection. Although this study noted the success in this single patient it also emphasized the impractical nature of providing this type of cure due to the invasive nature of total bone marrow ablation. In contrast, the researchers found that autologous transplantation of genetically altered CD4 cells which had been modified through disabling C-C chemokine receptor type 5 (CCR5), which is the main co-receptor utilized by HIV-1 for cell infection was both more effective and practical (Ye, et al., 2014).

Study Three: RNA-directed gene editing specifically eradicates latent and prevents new HIV-1 infection (July, 2014)

This study conducted by researchers Hu, Kaminski, Yang, Zhang, Consenting, Li…Khalili (2014) focused on new strategies to safely and effectively cleave HIV from host cells post infection and prevent reinfection utilizing a Cas9/guided RNA (gRNA) system. Study researchers additionally emphasized the elimination of; virus integration, viral gene expression, viral replication, latent reservoir strongholds, genotoxicity and off-target editing. HIV is a worldwide health problem with an infected population of approximately thirty-five million people (Maartens, Celum & Lewin, 2015). As a result of this worldwide impact, researchers have been working to develop new approaches to battle HIV. Gene editing is one such approach.

The RNA-directed gene editing study utilized the pre-existing, bacteria based, defense mechanism known as clustered regularly interspaced short palindromic repeats (CRISPR), associated 9 (Cas9) that researchers assert has demonstrated promise for targeting and eliminating HIV from host cells. According to researchers, one of the driving forces of this study's approach was to disrupt cell entry of HIV at numerous possible gateways via introduction of genetically modified CRISPR/Cas9 and other engineered biologic elements that have demonstrated specific and previously unseen abilities to hinder infection (Hu, et al., 2014).

Chapter Summary

HIV and AIDS continue to be critical health problems here in the U.S. and globally with millions of new cases diagnosed each year. The worldwide nature of the disease is one factor that prompts researchers to search for a vaccine and a cure. "The pandemic caused by the human immunodeficiency virus type 1 (HIV-1) is now in its fourth decade, with an estimated 2.5 million new infections occurring annually worldwide" (Hammer, et al., 2013). Recent months have provided promising scientific breakthroughs that could end the epidemic. For example, the discoveries of CRISPR/Cas9 and genetic therapies for the first time allow researchers to literally erase HIV from a living host cell. This discovery allows the immune system to return to normal as if the virus was never present and it prevents future infection from occurring through immunity. Other encouraging discoveries from geneticists such as TALENS could also play a part in eradicating the virus (Ye, et al., 2014).

Will a vaccine for HIV effectively prevent the transmission of HIV? Research studies have been conducted in the hopes of answering this very question. Studies such as those that have been included here provide information regarding how HIV mutates and means by which researchers may possibly develop an effective vaccine. The LTFU study demonstrates research efforts in examining the efficacy and safety of potential HIV vaccines in human subjects. Additional studies, both study two and three above, demonstrated potentially valuable information regarding the possibility of safely cleaving HIV from living cells as well as preventing future infection.

Due to the fact that HIV and AIDS have remained a health crisis for so many years, many people still want information on new research discoveries that could be utilized to eliminate HIV from a person already infected. Only a single person to-date is thought to have been cured of the infection. His name is Timothy Brown and he is known as "The Berlin Patient". His immune system was totally obliterated in the process of treating him for Leukemia. Once destroyed, his immune system was rebuilt utilizing genetically modified, HIV resistant, CD4 and CD8 cells that retained their ability to replicate. Due to the complexity and high probability of death associated with the treatment in Mr. Brown's case; it is impractical to repeat this on a large scale although it has been repeated in a controlled laboratory setting (Pelletier, 2015).

The new genetic modeling approaches, such as CRISPR/Cas9, in combination with TALENS, are beginning to tip the balance in favor of being able to actually eliminate the HIV/AIDS virus from individuals already infected by HIV. (Hu, et al., 2014). There is much work yet to be done in order to overcome challenges, such as off-target editing and mutation that currently pose serious health risks for human subjects, but the studies above suggest researchers are progressing toward that very goal.

If the answers to the two prior questions both prove to be positive, will the combination of the two effectively end the HIV epidemic? The theory of combination has long been an integral part of fighting HIV and AIDS. For example, combination drug regimens utilize multiple compounds to effectively debilitate the virus at multiple points of the infection cycle thus slowing disease progression. "Combination antiretroviral therapy (cART) for HIV infection has improved immune function and reduced the burden of opportunistic infections, prolonging survival for HIV-infected individuals in the United States" (Kowalkowski, Mims & Du, 2014). This same "combination" train of thought parallels the course that many researchers are pursuing. For the first time, researchers can now effectively remove the virus from host cells and provide immunity. The discoveries discussed above are individually relevant in their own right. However, when we combine discoveries of different groups of researchers and scientists are we able to see progress towards an end to HIV and AIDS?

Chapter 4: Results

Purpose of The Study

This mixed-method, qualitative study was conducted in order to assess how close the research community is to perfecting a vaccine and other methods to eradicate HIV from and infected person. More specifically this study investigated; (A) if an effective vaccine was in development and (B) if other means of eradicating the virus from an already infected person exist. Further, if both (A) and (B) are positive would that result in (C) the end of the HIV pandemic? Three studies were reviewed for the purpose of answering these three questions. Many vaccines have been studied over the last three decades in the fight against the disease. However, only the most recent trials were included here as they represent the most current approach and thinking toward a vaccine. Study one examines follow-up of clinical trial patients for five different vaccines and vaccine combinations (a vaccine plus a booster [see Key Terms Definitions]). This study illustrated the understanding by researchers that the traditional approach of a single, broad spectrum vaccine would be ineffective against HIV. As a result of this concept, this study demonstrated researchers shifted their approach to using vaccines in combination in order to increase longer-lasting immune system response. Study two researchers focused on a completely different research approach to imparting immunity.

This study's focus was on recreating natural immunity which has been found in a very small percentage of the population found to have a specific genetic mutation. Researchers were successful in recreating this genetic mutation in a laboratory setting. In the third study researchers concentrated on an even more progressive approach to the disease. The researchers successfully utilized the bacterial defense mechanism (in a genetically modified form) to achieve a dual effect, both eradiation of HIV from an infected person and imparting permanent immunity.

The research questions asked were;

1. Will a vaccine for HIV effectively prevent the transmission of HIV?

2. Are there any new research discoveries that could potentially be used to eliminate HIV from an infected person?

3. If the first two questions prove positive, will the combination of the two answers effectively end the HIV epidemic?

From these questions the following hypotheses are created;

H1a: Those vaccinated for HIV are more likely to become infected with HIV.

H10: Those vaccinated for HIV are less likely to become infected with HIV.

H2a: It is likely that there are new research discoveries that could potentially be utilized to eliminate HIV from a person already infected.

H20: It is not likely that there are new research discoveries that could potentially be utilized to eliminate HIV from a person already infected.

H3a: If the answers to the first two questions prove positive, the combination of the two is likely to effectively end the HIV epidemic.

H30: If the answers to the first two questions prove positive, the combination of the two is unlikely to effectively end the HIV epidemic.

This chapter provides detailed data results of each of the studies utilized in this secondary study. Following each set of written descriptive statistics there will be graphs, tables and charts to provide additional illustrative clarity of study findings. This chapter also concludes with a brief overview of the data presented in the Summary of Findings.

Descriptive Statistics

Study One: Long-term Follow-up (LTFU) of Study Participants from Prophylactic HIV Vaccine Clinical Trials in Africa (2014)

In these observational study researchers Schmidt et al., (2014), followed 287 volunteer participants from a larger, Phase I and II HIV preventive vaccine trial conducted between 2001 and 2007 in African countries. One of the prime areas of focus was the assessment of persistent vaccine-induced immune response, a positive indicator of vaccine effectiveness. The long-term effects of five different vaccines were evaluated; two separate recombinant plasmid DNA vaccines and three viral vector vaccines.

Post follow up in the respective initial vaccine trial, LTFU study participation was offered to both vaccine and placebo recipients. There was no difference in vaccine to placebo ratio of volunteers who were enrolled in the LTFU versus the original vaccine trial. The participant pool was comprised of 69 female and 153 male vaccine recipients and 22 female and 43 male placebo recipients. The following graph is illustrative of the gender demographics of the participant pool;

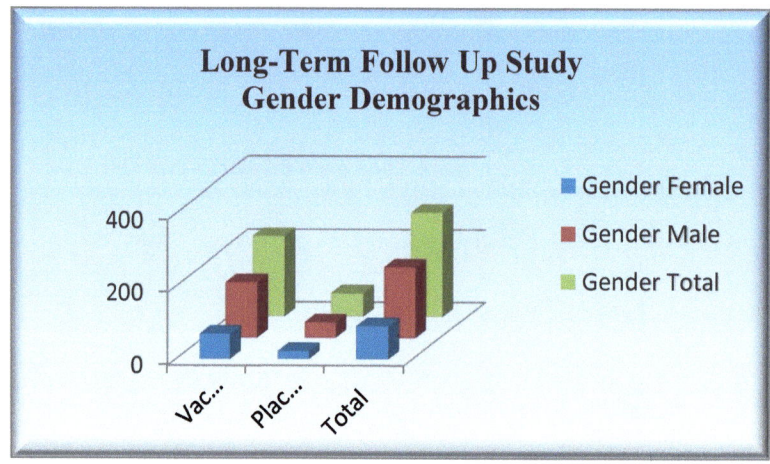

Table 1

Amongst LTFU study participants, six acquired HIV subsequent to the last dosage they received; one of the 65 placebo recipients and five of the 222 vaccine recipients. The time frame from final vaccination/placebo to diagnosis ranged from 11-64 months.

The Long-term Follow up (LTFU) study of the five potential vaccines was designed to elicit an immune response effectively triggering prolonged HIV immunity. The vaccines studied were all based on strains of the virus that are prevalent in the geographic region of Africa. Two different testing mechanisms were used throughout the study, the Capillus (Rapid) test and the Murex (ELISA) test. Researchers found that although the Rapid test is adequate for general population testing it was not as sensitive as the ELISA test. The ELISA, acronym for enzyme linked immune-sorbent assay, test is the predominant and preferred testing method known due to its heightened sensitivity to HIV antibodies present in an infected person (over the more expedient but less sensitive Rapid test). The LTFU study was conducted in six different countries over an eight year period. The following flow chart follows enrollees through the study process;

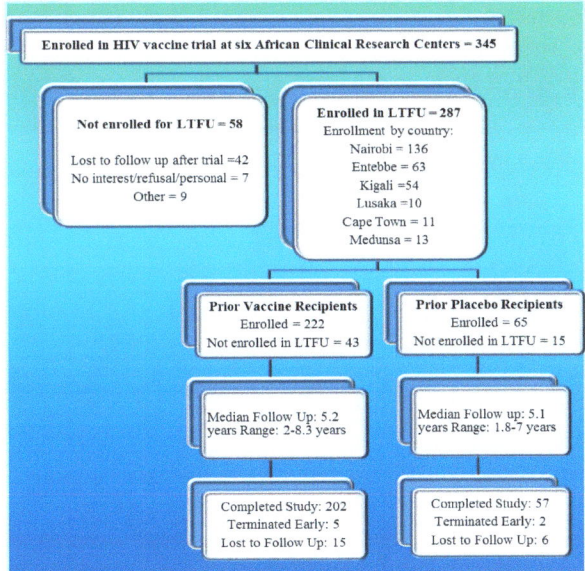

Table 2

There were three study participants who received vaccines during the original vaccine trial but had no detectable vaccine-induced antibodies during those trials. These three participants subsequently tested positive for HIV during the LTFU study indicating some vaccine-induced antibodies well after their last dosage; 4.5 years, 2.5 years and 3 years respectively. Subsequent testing revealed none of the three individuals to be HIV positive.

The study noted that due to a growing number of prophylactic HIV vaccine trials which utilize healthy, HIV negative volunteer participants, the prevalence of vaccine induced sero-reactivity (VISR) is increasing. Presence of VISR renders a false positive HIV test result due to detectable vaccine induced antibodies. However the occurrence of the false positive tests depends upon factors such as test sensitivity and the type and dosage of vaccine administered. There were insignificant reports of side effects, none of which were attributable to the vaccines in the trial.

Study Two: Seamless Modification of Wild-Type Induced Pluripotent Stem Cells to the Natural CCR5Δ32 Mutation Confers Resistance to HIV Infection

The researchers Ye, Wang, Beyer, Teque, Cradick, Qi, ... Kan, (2014), in this study sought to replicate the naturally occurring genetic mutation, C-C chemokine receptor type 5 genes with 32-bp deletions (CCR5Δ32), which provide natural HIV immunity to a small percentage of the human population. The researchers found that their hybrid strategy (combining PiggyBac technology and TALENS or CRISPR) exactly replicates this naturally occurring genetic characteristic while at the same time leaving no residual sequences within the genome they targeted. Residual sequences, or off-target mutations, have thus far proven to be a stumbling block for researchers due to the fact that this can lead to genetic abnormalities causing a range of health risks and problems, including death. This study categorically proves that, for the first time, through this hybrid method researchers are able to induce pluripotent stem cells (iPSCs) with the CCR5Δ32 mutation, effectively transferring immunity to a cell.

The findings in this study were; the effective means of creating a targeting construct which carries the 32-bp mutation [see CCR5Δ32 in Key Terms], the ability to excise the exact location where the natural CCR5Δ32 occurs and the ability to insert the new construct into the host genome at that location [see section A of the chart which follows this descriptive] (Ye, et al., 2014). Researchers in this study also found a near 100 percent success rate in targeting puromycin-resistant colonies in a single CCR5 allele utilizing TALEN pairs and PiggyBac technology, of which a 14 percent average was achieved in simultaneously targeting both alleles (Ye, et al., 2014). Puromycin resistant clones were picked and screened using Polymerase Chain Reaction (PCR) [see section B

of the chart which follows this descriptive] (Ye, et al., 2014).

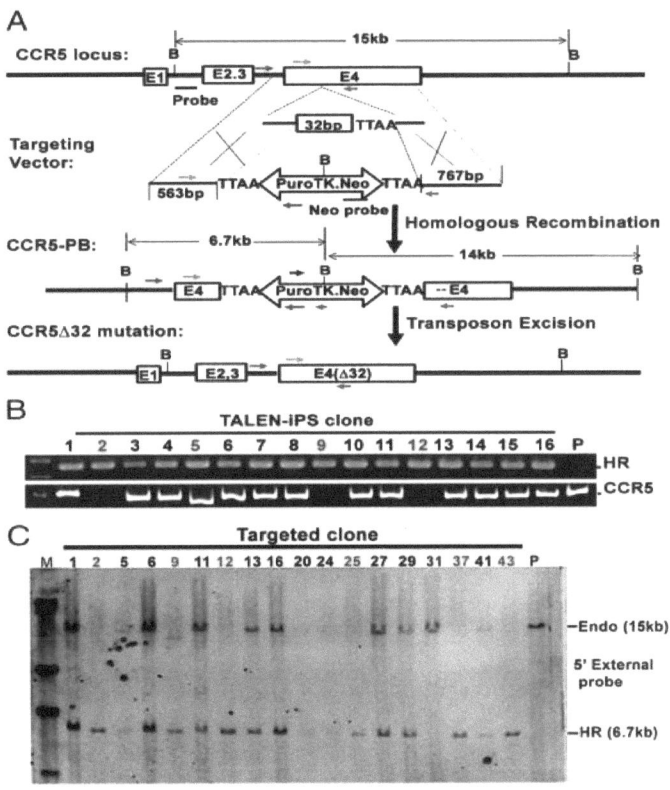

Table 3

According to researchers Ye, et al. (2014), use of a "…combination of double-

strand cleavage with TALENS or CRISPR/Cas9 and PiggyBac technology, with positive

and negative selections, methods generated biallelic Δ32 mutations precisely matching

the naturally occurring homozygous CCR5Δ32 genotype". Researchers further

elaborated that results demonstrated a near 100 percent efficiency of recombination for a

single allele as well as twenty-two and thirty-three percent for double alleles utilizing the

TALENS and RNA guided CRISPR/Cas9 approaches respectively.

Study Three: RNA-Directed Gene Editing Specifically Eradicates Latent and Prevents New HIV-1 Infection

Researchers Hu, et al (2014), in this mixed-methods study, assessed the ability of genetically modified guide RNAs (gRNAs) to seek out and kill proviral DNA from latently infected myeloid cells which operate as reservoirs, or hiding places for HIV. With current medications and treatments, as long as HIV remains dormant the virus is impervious to threat. However, the methods demonstrated within this study not only prove that latent HIV that is hidden within reservoirs can be forced to activate (making it vulnerable to medications) but also provide the host immunization against HIV-1 infection. Researchers found that their preventative vaccination is independent of HIV-1 strain's diversity due to the fact that the method specifies genomic sequences irrespective of how the virus entered the host cell.

This study by Hu, et al., confirmed that cells which stably expressed the Cas9/LTR-A/B effectively immunized TZM-bI cells from infection of HIV-1 [see figure A in the following illustration]. In the control (U6-CAG) HIV-1 infected cells are flagged in green while the subject cells on the right (Cas9/LTR-A/B genetically modified) remained immunized against infection after exposure to HIV-1 [see figures C and D in the following illustration] (2014).

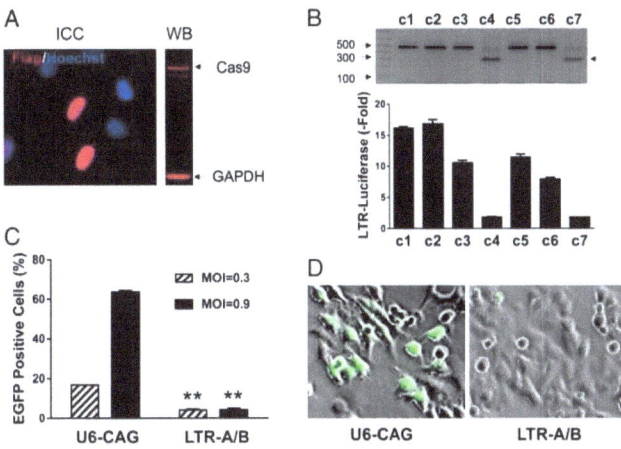

Table 4

The study scientists explained the demonstration of high specificity of

Cas9/gRNAs in editing the HIV-1 target genome. In other words, their method was both

highly exact and effective at cleaving the HIV-1 virus from the host cell which it has

infected and at the same time providing that host cell immunity against future infection.

This study effectively proved that HIV-1 can be eradicated from an infected cell through

genotyping for the purposes of developing personalized gene modification therapy for

individual patients. Researchers Hu, et al., (2014) asserted that the preexistence of the

Cas9/gRNA system in cells produced a quick elimination of new HIV-1 prior to it

infecting the host genome. The researchers compared this characteristic directly to the

bacterial defense system from which both Cas9 and CRISPR biotechnology were derived.

The research findings in this study reported that the Cas9/gRNA technology model was

swiftly progressing, was versatile and improving quickly toward clinical applications

specifically in the arenas of viral infection, genetic disorders and oncology treatment.

The research study found that the Cas9/gRNA model eliminated the HIV-1 genome and proficiently immunized targeted cells from HIV-1 infection with a high degree of efficacy, categorizing this as a possible means to a permanent HIV-1 cure.

Summary of Findings

The objective of this study was to determine whether or not a vaccine for HIV will effectively prevent the transmission of HIV, are there any new research discoveries that could be used to eliminate HIV from an infected person and if both of the questions are answered with a yes; will the combination of the two answers effectively end the HIV epidemic? The results of this study were very illuminating because great progress has been made in the fields of both HIV and Genetics. This study indicated that an effective vaccine for HIV can prevent infection and, thus transmission of the virus. However, the study also indicated that because HIV is a retrovirus the path to an effective vaccine will be different than for traditional viruses that research has prevailed over.

This study was also informative regarding the number of strains of HIV, how they most likely originated and entered the human population. This genetic lineage information could be critical in fighting HIV because understanding how the virus genetically mutates could provide the key to creating immunity within the human genome. Prime examples of this genetic linkage were the discoveries of CRISPR, Cas9 and TALEN biotechnologies which not only demonstrated ability to eradicate HIV-1 from cells but also served to provide permanent immunity from future HIV-1 infection.

Chapter five discusses the interpretations of research findings, implications for the research/medical communities and what these findings could mean in the fight against

HIV. Conclusions and recommendations for future studies and research are included at the end of chapter five.

Chapter 5: Introduction, Conclusion and Recommendations

Introduction

The purpose of this study was to address three key questions: Is a vaccine in development that is effective against HIV, a means for eradicating the virus from an already infected person in development? And if the answer to both of these questions is yes, does that mean we are close to the end of the pandemic? This study investigated these three questions through analysis of the history of HIV and its most likely origins, the genetic lineage of the virus and mutations, recent studies on potential vaccines and other progress in the field of HIV genetic therapies. This chapter will provide a brief overview of the information derived from studies and literature considered within this study, a conclusion based on the information and recommendations for future research. This chapter will conclude with a summary of this study.

Overview

It has long been said that knowledge is power. Early in the epidemic, after losing several close friends to the disease, I became motivated to understand more about what was killing my friends. At that time I did not know that I would lose many more friends over the ensuing years…many more than any young person should lose. Over twenty years ago I began working as an educator and advocate for those living with HIV and AIDS. I was a certified HIV/AIDS educator with the Monterey County Aids Project (MCAP) in Monterey, California. Just like the evolution of the research surrounding the disease, my knowledge has grown.

The HIV/AIDS pandemic is now in the thirty-fourth year and an estimated thirty-nine million people worldwide have died as a result of the infection ("UNAIDS fact sheet", 2015). Education programs for the public regarding safe sex practices, avoiding promiscuous behavior and refraining from sharing needles for intravenous drug users have been only marginally successful in curbing the spread of the disease. Advances in HIV pharmaceutical development have been far more successful in transforming the disease into more of a chronic condition rather than the death sentence the diagnosis was in the early to middle 1980's.

Although medications and treatments for the disease have vastly improved over this time both a vaccine and a cure have eluded researchers. Studies have shown that HIV is unlike other viruses because it is a retrovirus; meaning that traditional approaches to creating a vaccine are ineffective due to the virus's ability to quickly mutate. This has frustrated researchers and hampered their efforts in the search for a vaccine and a cure. However, this frustration has prompted the research community to seek unique approaches that are more effective against the virus.

Conclusions

Throughout the studies it was discovered that sometimes approaches do not work and, in many instances, the information could be just as important as a breakthrough that does work. This is definitely true concerning studies of vaccines for HIV. Numerous studies have proven that traditional vaccine development methodologies are not effective against HIV because it is a retrovirus and it mutates very quickly. Traditional vaccines are strain specific, and when a virus mutates a new strain is the result. This is one reason many vaccines for HIV have realized little success. The LTFU study by researchers

Schmidt, et al., (2014) demonstrated this lack of long-term immunity. However, this result has prompted researchers to explore new approaches to battling HIV and AIDS. In an effort to capitalize on the very small percentage of the population whose genetic makeup provides them natural immunity, researchers Ye, et al., (2014) have successfully replicated this genetic anomaly in a laboratory setting. In the findings of this second study, researchers created a hybrid approach (combining PiggyBac technology with either TALENS or CRISPR) in order to precisely replicate natural immunity. Approaching HIV/AIDS research from "outside the box" is increasingly yielding positive results. For example in the third study, researchers Hu, et al., (2014) have, for the first time, harnessed the defense mechanism of bacteria and are modifying it to both cleave HIV from an infected cell and replace the viral material with immunity. This study was particularly insightful because not only were researchers successful at genetically modifying gRNAs to seek out and kill latent HIV but their method simultaneously imparts immunization against HIV-1 infection.

In light of these studies, the information impacts the research questions in the following ways;

1. Will a vaccine for HIV effectively prevent the transmission of HIV?

Based on the studies included herein the most likely answer to this question is yes, once it is developed and perfected. However, a vaccine for HIV is also likely to be very unlike any vaccine that we know to date. Also based on this research, immunization may be derived from genetically modified bacterial defense systems such as CRISPR, Cas9 and TALENS. These gene modification based biotechnologies have proven successful in laboratory testing in mice but must be translated into a form which would be efficacious for use in people.

2. Are there any new research discoveries that could potentially be used to eliminate HIV from an infected person?

Once again, this study demonstrates that there are indeed new discoveries that could be used for this purpose. Both study two and three demonstrated different methodologies which were successful at achieving this in the respective laboratory settings.

3. If questions 1 and 2 prove positive, will the combination of the two answers effectively end the HIV epidemic?

In theory, for the purposes of this academic argument, yes that should be enough to end the HIV epidemic. A positive answer to both questions one and two would theoretically provide the knowledge required to end the HIV/AIDS epidemic. However, limitations beyond the scope of this study could delay or prevent realization of a complete end to the existence of the disease.

Limitations of This Study

Numerous limitations to this study exist; some are identifiable and some are not. Known potential limitations include politics, social, moral, religious, geographic and even financial elements…any one of (or combination of) which could preclude the end of the epidemic. Political struggles of under developed, war-torn nations could prevent immunization even if a perfect vaccine is developed. Fear of vaccination, social, moral and religious beliefs could result in some people refusing immunization even if it is made available at no cost. Finally, particularly in today's economically driven pharmaceutical market; a cure for such a widespread disease would likely be worth an untold fortune.

Ownership of a vaccine or treatment would likely pose serious ethical issues for any entity that proposes withholding supply for payment. Costly treatments are out of reach for poor and clinically underserved populations globally. The processes of mass production and distribution will likely also present a host of challenges.

Recommendations for Future Research

Development of unique approaches (or combinations of approaches) to fighting HIV/AIDS should be studied. Future studies should be conducted regarding how to overcome obstacles to vaccination and treatment including; socio-economic and vaccination fear. Research should also be conducted to explore the possibility of treatments rather than relying solely on pharmaceutical remedies (i.e. radiation in oncology). In conclusion, while this will require research, preparation should be made to begin manufacturing and distribution of the vaccine/treatment/medication as soon as it is available; to the U.S. and globally.

References

Aids research alliance (2015). Our progress in developing prostratin: From hope to cure.

Retrieved from http://aidsresearch.org/cure-research/our-progress

Avert: HIV and aids science (2015). History of HIV up to 1986. Retrieved from

http://www.avert.org/hiv-and-aids-science.htm

Barclay, S. L., Yang, Y., Zhang, S., Fong, R., Barraza, A., Nolta, J. A. … & Anderson, J.

S. (2015). Safety and efficacy of a tCD25 preselective combination Anti-HIV

Lentiviral vector in human hematopoietic stem and progenitor cells. STEM

CELLS, 33: 870–879. doi: 10.1002/stem.1919

Bird, J. & Voisin, D. (2013). "You're an open target to be abused": A qualitative study of

stigma and HIV self-disclosure among black men who have sex with men.

American Journal of Public Health. 103(12), 2193-2199.

Birnbaum, J. K., Murray, C. J. L., & Lozano, R. (2011). Exposing misclassified

HIV/AIDS deaths in South Africa. World Health Organization.Bulletin of the

World Health Organization, 89(4), 278-85. Retrieved from

https://search.proquest.com/docview/863441560?accountid=41759

Bernstein, M. (2015). New lead against HIV could finally hobble the virus's edge.

Medical Express, Retrieved from http://medicalxpress.com/news/2015-03-hiv-

hobble-virus-edge.html

Cohen, M. S., Smith, M. K., Muessig, K. E., Hallet, T. B., Powers, K. A., & Kashuba, A.

D. (2013). Antiretroviral treatment of hiv-1 prevents transmission of hiv-1: Where do we go from here? The Lancet, 382(9903), 1515-1524. doi:

http://dx.doi.org/10.1016/S0140-6736(13)61998-4

Deeks, S. G., Lewin, S. R., & Havlir, D. V. (2013). The end of aids: Hiv infection as a

chronic disease. The Lancet, 382(9903), 1525-1533. doi:

http://dx.doi.org/10.1016/S0140-6736(13)61809-7

Doudna, J. A. (2015). Genomic engineering and the future of medicine. JAMA, 313(8),

791. Retrieved from

https://search.proquest.com/docview/1660922793?accountid=41759

Ebina, H., Misawa, N., Kanemura, Y., & Koyanagi, Y. (2013). Harnessing the crispr/cas9

system to disrupt latent hiv-1 provirus: Scientific reports. Nature, 3, doi:

10.1038/srep02510

France, L. R. (2011, March 23). Elizabeth taylor championed aids charity passionately.

CNN news. Retrieved from

http://www.cnn.com/2011/SHOWBIZ/03/23/elizabeth.taylor.charity.work/index.h

tml

Francis, D. P. (2012). Deadly AIDS policy failure by the highest levels of the US

government: A personal look back 30 years later for lessons to respond better to

future epidemics. Journal of Public Health Policy, 33(3), 290-300.

doi:http://dx.doi.org/10.1057/jphp.2012.14

Giordano, T. P. (2015). The HIV treatment cascade-a new tool in HIV prevention. The

Journal of the American Medical Association, Retrieved from

http://amaprod.silverchaircdn.com/data/Journals/INTEMED/0/iic140090.pdf.gif?

v=635600531395400000

Hammer, S. M., Sobieszczyk, Magdalena E., Janes, H., Karuna, S. T., Mulligan, M. J., Grove, D... & Gilbert, P. B. (2013). Efficacy trial of a DNA/rAd5 HIV-1 preventive vaccine. *The New England Journal of Medicine.* 369(22), 2083-92. Retrieved from

https://search.proquest.com/docview/1462420360?accountid=41759

Hosein, S. R. (2015). British Columbia researchers examine past and future directions in the HIV epidemic. The Body Pro: The HIV Resource for Health Professionals, Retrieved from http://www.thebodypro.com/content/75561/british-columbia-researchers-examine-past-and-futu.html?getPage=2

Hu, W., Kaminski, R., Yang, F., Zhang, Y., Cosentino, L., Li, F. … Khalili, K. (2014). RNA-directed gene editing specifically eradicates latent and prevents new HIV-1 infection. Proceedings of the National Academy of Sciences of the United States of America, 111(31), 11461–11466. doi:10.1073/pnas.1405186111

Kempner, M. (2015). Why HIV vaccines may be failing. The Body Pro: The HIV Resource for Health Professionals, Retrieved from http://www.thebodypro.com/content/75406/why-hiv-vaccines-may-be-failing.html?ic=wnhp

Kempner, M. (2015). With HIV care as the goal, gene therapy research expands. The Body: The complete hiv/aids resource, Retrieved from http://www.thebody.com/content/75612/with-hiv-cure-as-the-goal-gene-therapy-research-ex.html?ic=wnhp

Kowalkowski, M. A., Mims, M. A., Day, R. S., Du, X. L., Chan, W., & Chiao, E. Y. (2014). Longer duration of combination antiretroviral therapy reduces the risk of hodgkin lymphoma: A cohort study of HIV-infected male veterans. Cancer

Epidemiology, 38(4), 386-92. doi:http://dx.doi.org/10.1016/j.canep.2014.05.009

Lahey, T. P. (2015). So much has changed since the first HIV test was approved 30 years

ago. *Medical Express.* Retrieved from http://medicalxpress.com/news/2015-03-

hiv-years.html

Laurence, M.D., J. (2015). Boosting killer t cells to eliminate HIV reservoirs. Amfar

making aids history, Retrieved from http://www.amfar.org/Early-ART-and-

Boosting-Immuning/

Lovell, S. A., & Rosenberg, M. W. (2011). Community capacity amongst people living

with HIV/AIDS. *GeoJournal.* 76(2), 111-121.

doi:http://dx.doi.org/10.1007/s10708-009-9289-2

Maartens, G., Celum, C., & Lewin, S. R. (2014). HIV infection: Epidemiology,

pathogenesis, treatment, and prevention. The Lancet, 384(9939), 258-71.

doi:http://dx.doi.org/10.1016/S0140-6736(14)60164-1

Martlett, J., Belmonte, J. C. I., Liao, H., Esteban, C., Hishida, T., Takahashi, Y., & Li, M.

(2015). Cellular scissors chop up hiv virus. Med Express, Retrieved from

http://medicalxpress.com/news/2015-03-cellular-scissors-hiv-virus.html

McNeil, D. (2015, February 19). New approach to blocking hiv raises hopes for aids

vaccine. The New York Times. Retrieved from

http://www.nytimes.com/2015/02/19/health/new-approach-to-blocking-hiv-raises-

talk-of-an-aids-vaccine.html?_r

Namuleme, R., Ford, N., & Bath, P. (2015). Information disconnects for people infected

with, or affected by, hiv/aids in the United Kingdom. Direct Research Journal of

Social Sciences and Educational Studies. 2nd, 38-44. Retrieved from

http://www.directresearchpublisher.org/drjsses/archive/2015/Feb/PDF/Namuleme

et al.pdf

National Institute of Health, National Institute of Allergy and Infectious Disease. (2015).

HIV vaccine research. Retrieved from website:

http://www.niaid.nih.gov/topics/hivaids/research/vaccines/Pages/default.aspx

Pelletier, S., Gingras, S., & Green, D. R. (2015). Mouse genome engineering via

CRISPR-Cas9 for study of immune function. Immunity, 42(1), 18-27.

doi:http://dx.doi.org/10.1016/j.immuni.2015.01.004

Picker LJ, Hansen SG, Lifson JD. New Paradigms for HIV/AIDS Vaccine Development.

Annual Review of Medicine. 2012; 63:95-111. doi:10.1146/annurev-med-

042010-085643.

Schmidt, C., Jaoko, W., Omosa-Manyonyi, G., Kaleebu, P., Mpendo, J., Nanvubya, A …

Fast, P. E. (2014). Long-term follow-up of study participants from prophylactic

HIV vaccine clinical trials in Africa. Human Vaccines & Immunotherapeutics,

10(3), 714–723. doi:10.4161/hv.27559

Sharp, P., & Hahn, B. (2011). Origins of HIV and the aids pandemic. Cold spring harbor

perspectives in medicine, doi: 10.1101/cshperspect.a006841

Stover, G. N. & Northridge, Mary E. (2013). The social legacy of HIV/AIDS. *American

Journal of Public Health* 103(2), 199. Retrieved from

https://search.proquest.com/docview/1312687629?accountid=41759

Tachikawa, R., Tomii, K., Murase, K., Ueda, H., Harada, Y., Kida, Y., & Ishihara, K.

(2011). Therapeutic effect of direct hemoperfusion with a polymyxin Bimmobilized fiber column in the treatment of HIV-negative severe pneumocystis pneumonia. Respiration, 81(4), 318-24. doi:http://dx.doi.org/10.1159/000316340

United Nations AIDS programme, (2015). Unaids fact sheet. Retrieved from the United Nations website: Unknown, A. (2015, March 29). Unaids fact sheet Retrieved from

http://www.unaids.org/en/resources/campaigns/2014/2014gapreport/factsheet

U.S. Military, HIV Research Program. (2015). Thai phase iii HIV vaccine clinical trial rv144. Retrieved from http://www.hivresearch.org/research.php?ServiceID=13

Ye, L., Wang, J., Beyer, A. I., Teque, F., Cradick, T. J., Qi, Z. … Kan, Y. W. (2014). Seamless modification of wild-type induced pluripotent stem cells to the natural CCR5Δ32 mutation confers resistance to HIV infection. Proceedings of the National Academy of Sciences of the United States of America, 111(26), 9591–9596. doi:10.1073/pnas.1407473111

Zablotska, I. B., Holt, M., & Prestage, G. (2012). Changes in gay men's participation in gay community life: Implications for HIV surveillance and research. AIDS and behavior. 16(3), 669-75. doi:http://dx.doi.org/10.1007/s10461-011-9919-9

Tables

Table 1.

Long-Term Follow Up Study Gender Demographics

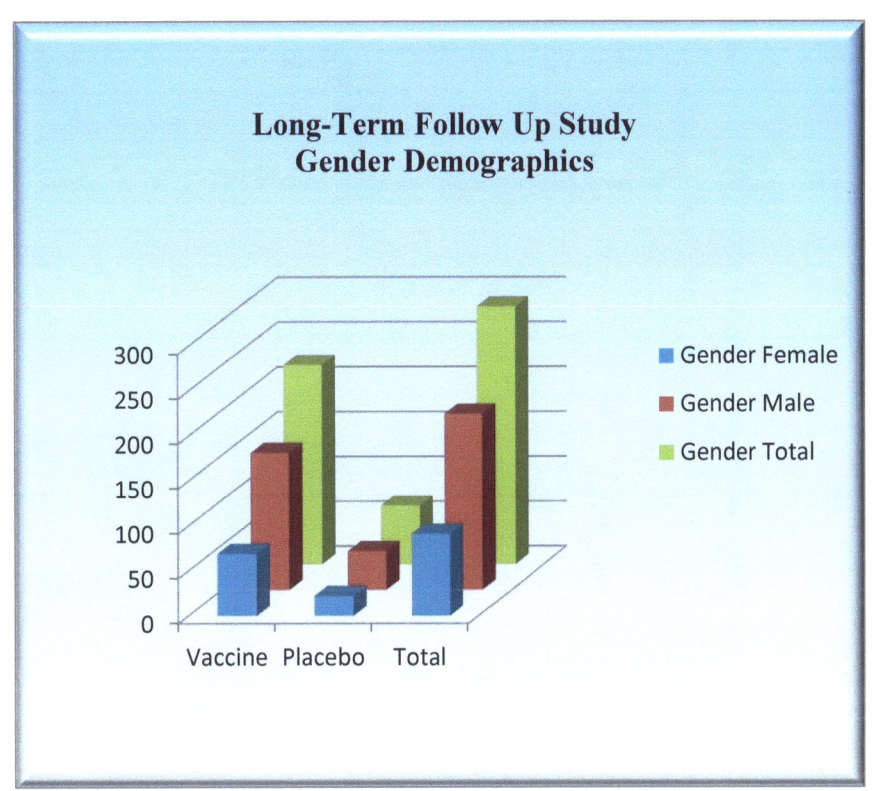

Table 2.

Enrollment in HIV Vaccine Trial at Six African Clinical Research Centers

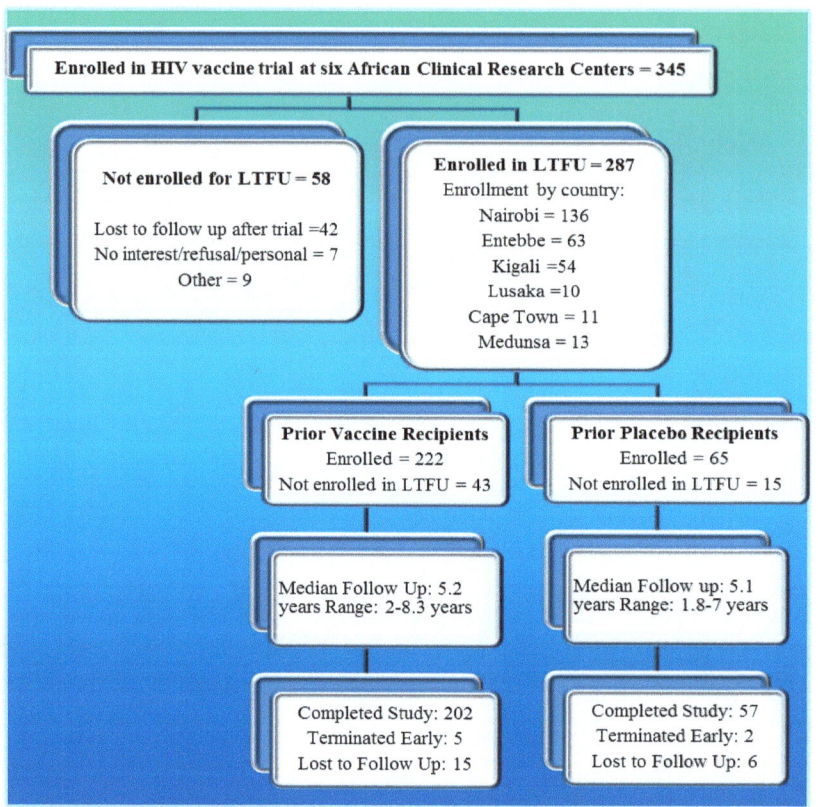

Table 3.

Laboratory Results Demonstrating CCR5Δ32 Replication

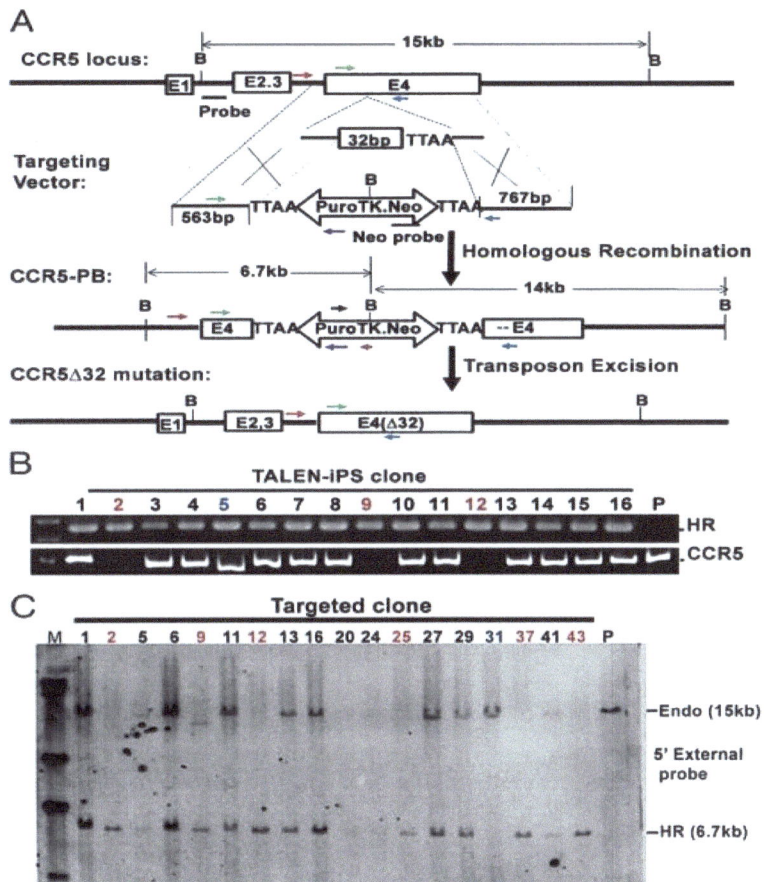

Table 4.

Laboratory Results Demonstrating RNA-Directed Gene Editing Eradication of Latent

HIV and Prevention of New Infection

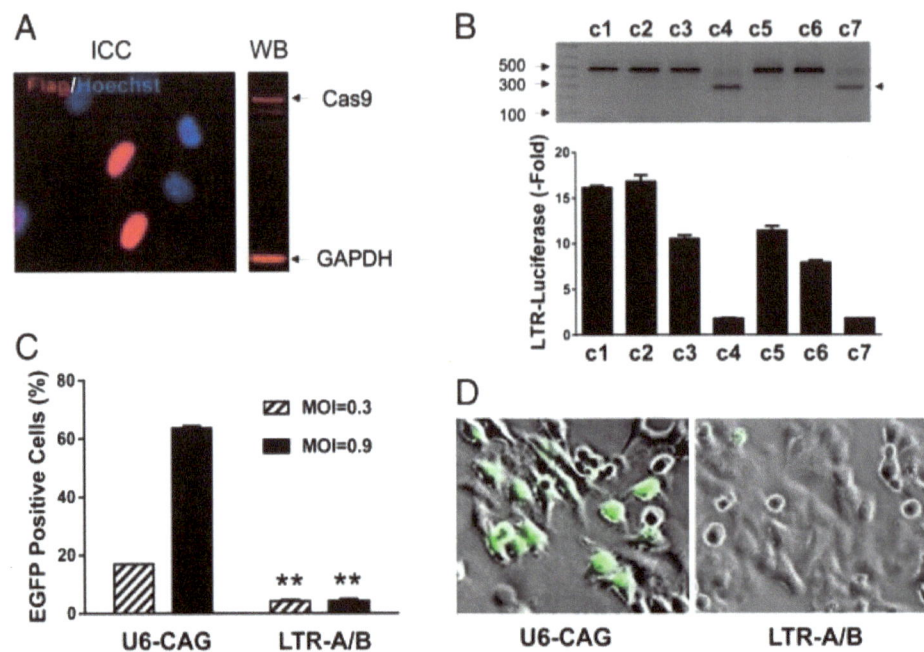

Appendices

Certificate of Completion

The National Institutes of Health (NIH) Office of Extramural Research certifies that **Michael Capristo** successfully completed the NIH Web-based training course "Protecting Human Research Participants".

Date of completion: 04/29/2015

Certification Number: 1752551

www.ingramcontent.com/pod-product-compliance
Lightning Source LLC
Chambersburg PA
CBHW050750180526
45159CB00003B/1406